INTERMITTENT FASTING FOR HEALTHY WEIGHT LOSS

Kitty Browne

Table of Contents

Meet the Caveman

In the days of the caveman, the idea of dieting was simply unheard of. Your average caveman didn't really think in terms of Caloric Restriction and Resting Metabolic Rate.

No, Thag the Caveman ate what he could, when he could.

Thag's problem wasn't an expanding waistline or an inflating cholesterol count. Thag didn't measure his blood pressure, didn't check his blood sugar, and he sure didn't stand in front of any mirrors.

Thag's problem was much simpler than that; he couldn't always get food. Oh, sure; if you could manage to hit the bison with the spear just right you had all kinds of food.

Until the meat went bad. Thag didn't even know how to salt his meat, let alone coat it in chemical preservatives. What he did know was that his bison had a clock ticking on it as soon as it hit the ground.

So Thag did the natural thing; he ate what he could when it was presented to him. And he would eat as much of that bison as he possibly could because, well, hunting bison is really hard. He had no idea where his next meal would come from, but he had food now and he knew what to do with it.

Now, this is a pretty simplified scenario. After all, there were cavemen all over, and they had varied survival techniques. Anthropologists may forgive me my Gary-Larson-like oversimplification, but the one thing all of those survival techniques had in common was this: all of them were luck-dependent. Whether you could hunt that bison or find that camas root, you needed to get lucky.

And you couldn't get lucky all the time.

As a result, prehistoric people spent most of their lives in famine, with brief periods of feast. The ones whose bodies could tolerate those kinds of pressures lived longer; the ones that could not would die out. Over the course of thousands of years, the Darwinian hand of natural selection pruned these proto-humans.

So why do we care about the hardships of Thag and his caveman kin? Well, Thag could very well be the great (times several hundred) grandfather of any of us, and his genes live on today in our bodies.

That system, plucked, pruned, and finely honed over thousands of years of natural selection, now resides in our modern bodies. Where we have been taught since birth to feed it three square meals a day.

These meals are ones we retrieve from the supermarket, or we head to a restaurant. We do not have to chase a bison down, or hunt through the plains for the right plant. It's just there, price sticker on, and we trade bits of paper or, even more arcane, bits of data on a magnetic-stripped card for them. We've given them names and calendared them into our daily work breaks. We mix spices from the Indian subcontinent with produce from the tropics and grains from the temperate zones.

Thag did not need a recipe for his food; he was pretty advanced if he cooked over fire at all.

If Thag could see the nonchalance with which we simply rise from our desks during the noon hour and declare it time for lunch, he would be flabbergasted. The idea that one could avoid famine simply by scheduling one's meals would, to a small caveman brain, be simply overwhelming.

Now, scientists have been studying Thag's diet. They have been studying the digestive system, our system, that Thag's diet produced. And they have come to a theory that should probably be less shocking than it is: Thag's digestive system is just as overwhelmed by our eating schedule as Thag's brain would have been.

Our digestive system was designed, laboriously, for feast and famine. It is built to harvest energy, store that energy, and then use that energy in the times we cannot feed again. Our cardiovascular system, lymphatic system, and excretory systems are all designed to service the energy and waste produced by this digestive system, and all evolved around the feast/famine dynamic.

We simply did not evolve on three square meals a day; the idea that three meals is the healthiest option now is a cultural, not a scientific, conclusion.

So now we look to alternatives. While we still do not need to chase down bison, "intermittent fasting" as a dieting technique is designed to emulate Thag's eating patterns. We give our system what it was designed for; larger amounts of food followed by little or no caloric intake in between. The specific effects of intermittent fasting are still being researched, but there have been a number of noticeable health benefits to the technique. It is called, by some, a "new diet." If Thag spoke English, he would disagree.

In reading this book, you will learn what science knows about intermittent fasting. We will explore the potential benefits, and potential hardships, of the technique. In the end, we may even help you expand your lifespan by reaching back through the mists of history and consuming your food in this most ancient of ways.

How Does I.F. Work?

So, why does intermittent fasting work? Well, given the number of different benefits to living like Thag, there's actually a number of different factors that go into the health benefits of this diet plan.

Let's break them apart, and look at them one by one.

Weight Loss

This one goes front and center because it is, invariably, the thing we are most concerned about.

Every one of us has a Resting Metabolic Rate. We are constantly maintaining brain function, breathing, and pumping blood through all of our organs. Our cells are constantly burning caloric value to produce heat. The number of calories burnt this way varies from person to person, and is dependent on your current weight and your level of activity in a day, which means we can raise our RMR by exercising.

When we consume more calories than our RMR, our body stores excess calories in the most efficient way it knows how; by producing fat. When we haven't fed our RMR enough, it burns that fat instead, using the stored energy to keep us alive.

This, of course, is the basics behind *any* diet plan; lower one's caloric intake and force the RMR to burn fat. Whether it be by cutting out carbohydrates (thus taking away those calories), low-fat diets (thus removing the stored calories of *other* organisms from our own diet), or the ubiquitous caloric restriction (CR) diets, the purpose is to make sure that you do not consume more calories than your RMR can burn.

Intermittent fasting does the same thing; by simply skipping eating for a period of time one skips the caloric intake of that time frame, thus reducing caloric intake. Pretty simple, right?

So why the heck do it this way? Caloric restriction diets are hard enough, right? I mean, we always feel hungry when we're cutting back on calories. There's that voice in the back of our head that tells us to get some more food *fast,* because *you are going to die of hunger,* right? That little, niggling demon of a voice constantly chats at you when you're eating during the day; how much worse, then, when you simply *stop* eating for a day?

And here's when we get into the really nifty science. Remember Thag; he ate what he could, when he could. If Thag kills a bison, Thag eats his bison. And he's happy about it. There's a reason for that. Food tends to make us hungry.

That's right, food makes us hungry. The very existence of food triggers a desire in the body to eat food; the brain releases a set of chemicals called (collectively) endorphins. They give us a sense of pleasure and happiness in eating, and they encourage us to eat more.

Four to five hours after we get that endorphin rush, it wears off. We come down off our high like a heroin junkie with no money. And it hurts, too. Our body *knows* what it needs to do to get those endorphins back; keep eating. So our body sends signals to our brain; eat something. Those signals are interpreted as hunger by our brains.

Simple caloric restriction diets play total havoc with this system. When you're on a Caloric Restriction diet, you are hitting your body with small doses of endorphins, then letting it dry out again.

In Greek mythology, Tantalus was a king who killed his infant son, then served him as a meal to the Gods. Horrified, the Gods refused to eat (with one exception, Demeter). For this heinous affront, Tantalus was given a powerful hunger and thirst. He was then stood in a cold, clear stream of water underneath an eternally ripe fruit tree. However, every time he tried to lower his lips to drink, the water would retreat from his lips. When he would reach for the fruit, it would remain eternally just barely out of his reach.

The Greek Gods were kind of jerks that way.

The point here is, a caloric restriction diet does *exactly this.* It gives the body a small taste of what the body *craves*, and then it cuts it off.

The body is constantly locked into a hunger cycle, forever keening its desires to the brain of the dieter. The food the dieter does eat serves the same function as Tantalus' stream and tree; it is little more than a prod to the deeper desires of the body. *Eat more,* our bodies tell us. *Eat until you cannot eat any more at all.* When we try eating only a little, we consistently prod our bodies into this response.

But here's the interesting thing; this kind of hunger, this hunger-as-drug-withdrawal, doesn't last. It's a powerful wave, but it comes, and then it goes.

And the going? Well, that's kind of the awesome part.

You see, our bodies are designed to reward us for eating; we all know that. Diet theory has been set up for *ages* to try to find creative workarounds for that powerful reward system. Our bodies are not, however, designed to permanently torment us for failing to eat. In fact, our bodies move past this psychologically-based hunger. We enter a state where our body has begun to…get this…*burn its reserves instead.* We stop feeling the dominant hunger craving.

That little, niggling voice in your head? It dies. You can, in fact, starve it to death without starving yourself. You won't feel full, but the powerful craving for food will subside into something much more complacent. Imagine how much less horrific Tantalus' punishment would be if he wasn't in that stream or under that tree.

After all, Thag couldn't be incapacitated; he had to be able to go hunt his next bison if he were going to survive. So it is with our bodies; we break past the point of withdrawal, and we go on with our lives.

Intermittent fasting is different from other forms of caloric restriction in that it takes advantage of this. You eat normally on one day, then go to sleep. By the time you rise in the morning, your 4-5 hour "hunger wave" window has passed. You've slept through your withdrawal; we do it every morning. You'll feel a little residual morning hunger, but not an overwhelming craving.

Then you drink some water, maybe some tea or some coffee, and go on with your day. You never trigger your endorphin rush, which means you never trigger your endorphin withdrawal, which means you avoid your cravings. The next day, you get up and eat normally.

Voila! Your total calorie count over those two days has been *cut in half,* while your cravings have been either killed (on a fast day) or fulfilled (on a feast day). Instead of constantly prodding your body with small amounts of food, you are maintaining your body in one of the two states it is used to dealing with: feast and famine. As a result, your body believes that all is normal, and ceases to send those annoying emergency claxons up to trigger your cravings.

The result of this is steady, consistent weight loss. Instead of wrestling with your willpower to avoid breaking into a binge (and we've all wrestled with that one), no wrestling match occurs. This prevents the old "diet rollercoaster" from ever leaving the station, which in turn leads to sustainable weight loss.

Human Growth Hormone

There are a lot of diets that promise weight loss. The question really comes around to what the side effects of those diets might be, and here's where intermittent fasting really shines.

To begin with, intermittent fasting forces the body to burn fat for extended periods of time. This is obvious, given that last section, but it's worth repeating. You see, in order to function solely off fat reserves, the body naturally produces somatotropin, more commonly known as the Human Growth Hormone (HGH). A 2007 study found an increase in HGH production of 1,300 percent in women, and nearly 2,000 percent in men over the course of a 24-hour fast.

Those are some pretty intense numbers, but they make sense. After all, the fast is forcing the body to shift solely into burn-fat mode, so it creates a whole bunch of the hormone that burns fat.

Now, researchers have long been arguing over the benefits of HGH supplements, and that's a fight that warrants a book (or several) on that subject alone. For our purposes, though, it doesn't matter; acclaim is nigh universal for HGH produced inside of our own bodies.

For instance, natural HGH can benefit production of cartilage in our joints. It can increases calcium retention, which strengthens our bones. It increases our muscle mass and increases our ability to synthesize proteins. It stimulates the growth and regeneration of all internal organs excluding the brain. It cranks up our immune system. And last but *certainly* not least, it reduces liver uptake of glucose, aids in gluconeogenesis in the liver, and buffs the living daylights out of our pancreatic islets, all of which helps regulate our blood sugar.

Remember, at the beginning of this chapter, we went over the basics of dieting. The goal, ultimately, is to consume fewer calories than one burns through one's

RMR. The beauty of HGH production as a result of one's *diet* is the boost to the RMR. This boost does not come as the result of a standard caloric restriction diet. As a result, even though the total caloric intake stays about the same between a normal caloric restriction diet and an intermittently fasting diet, the *gap* between calorie intake and RMR gets much larger when one intermittently fasts.

None of this should surprise us. When Thag was going into starvation mode, his body would be kicking itself into high gear, helping him build himself up so he could find his next food source. HGH was pumping through Thag, turning his fat reserves into muscle, cartilage, bone, and organ tissue. Thag's body turned itself into a killing machine, ready to find and consume his next prey.

When Thag fed, his body relaxed. It had food; it no longer needed to turn itself into a hunting/gathering machine. Thag's HGH levels plummeted.

Modern diets leave our HGH levels low. The only other thing that could comparably raise our HGH levels (outside of the controversial supplements) is high-intensity workouts. Modern diets never force our body to turn into lethal hunting machines; we never approach the primal glory that is Thag. Now that we understand what happens directly after our psychological hunger threshold, we know that an intermittent fasting diet can trigger that deep, primal part of us that wants to turn into a lethal machine, and put it to use improving our health instead.

You Have Options

Well, the basics of fasting are pretty easy: don't eat. That doesn't seem like it's a complicated procedure, right? After all, I've been talking about Caveman Thag this whole book, and it's not like he ever did anything complicated.

Of course, Thag really didn't have a choice.

He lived his life on the brink of starvation, constantly careening from one panicked moment to another. His life expectancy was maybe—*maybe*—twenty-five years. When we're talking about emulating Thag for a longer life, we probably need to pick and choose which parts of his diet to copy, not simply copy the whole lifestyle. At the end of the day, Thag's odds of outliving the modern lifespan were not the sort of thing you'd want to put money on.

You see, as we discussed in the previous chapter, as we fast our bodies begin burning our fat reserves in order to crank our systems up. The engine revs, getting the caveman ready to hunt his next bison.

The problem is this; our bodies turn into self-burning machines. And after not too long, they don't just burn fat. Our bodies will burn whatever they can to keep generating heat. Muscle mass, organ tissue; it all gets fed into the furnace hopper to keep us going. This is actual, physiological starvation. Unlike the psychological endorphin-withdrawal starvation we talked about last chapter, this kind of starvation presents a real risk to your health, and it is to be avoided.

So, the art to intermittent fasting isn't the *fasting*, it's the *intermittent.*

The idea is to put one's body in a fat-burning stage, but eat before it starts burning the rest of itself down. It's a game of chicken with starvation, trying to get as close as possible without going over the edge of the cliff.

Now, the simple thing to do here is to hand you a schedule: Fast on days X Y, Z… and eat on days A, B, and C.

No problem, right?

Huge problem. Your body and mine aren't calibrated exactly the same way. The intermittent fasting patterns that hold my body on that razor edge of the almost-starved vary from person to person. What works for me could very well trigger full starvation in you, or it may be too little to put your body into full-on HGH production. As a result, establishing the correct patterns for intermittent fasting is a very personal journey, and it's going to involve some trial and error.

In this chapter, we're going to establish how to go about that trial and error, to find the perfect balance point for your body.

The Twenty-Four Hour Fast

Your intermittent fasting is going to begin on a Saturday evening. Pick a time; 7:00 or 8:00 is fine, though some experts recommend going as late as 10:00pm. Whatever time you pick, eat at that time on Saturday. Make sure to hydrate. Then begin your fast.

During your fast, consume little to no calories. Water is encouraged, and if you take vitamin or protein supplements by all means continue doing so, but beyond that spend twenty-four hours not eating.

Sunday evening, at the same time you had dinner Saturday night, have a light snack (roughly 500 calories) to break your fast.

The goal here is to see how your body reacts to the fast. It's to demonstrate to your mind that it's OK to not eat for a decent chunk of time. It's also to gauge your body's reaction to the fast; at what points during the day did you feel good about what was happening, and at what points did you feel hunger cravings?

The trick here is to stay busy. Make sure your mind is focused on something *other* than the fact you aren't eating. If the hunger pangs really start to get to you at a certain time, make note of it, but don't spend the day *thinking* about not eating, or you'll have put yourself back into Tantalus' stream. Instead, make sure that you have plenty to do that Sunday.

By the end of your twenty-four hour fast, you'll have a pretty good idea what fasting feels like to you. Then, on Monday, resume a normal eating schedule, but *do not binge.* If you feel an overwhelming desire to binge, then you know that the longer fasting periods are not for you. If, however, you feel awake and energetic on Monday, then you know that you're going to be looking for those longer fasting periods, because they work for you.

As other experts do, I'm dividing fasting schedules up into what I've termed "long fasting" and "short fasting." One is not necessarily better than the other, but your twenty-four hour fast should have given you an idea which of these categories you're in. After that, it's just a matter of dialing in your specific pattern.

The Long Fast

The long fast is a fast that is twenty-four to thirty-six hours in length.

Never—and this is an ironclad rule here—*never* exceed thirty-six hours in a fast. You're not Ghandi trying to make a point, you're just a normal person trying to get a better body.

Thirty-six hours sounds like a long time, but if you were to completely not eat for a full daylight cycle, you would have the preceding and following night cycles to round out a full thirty-six hours. Going over that limit is *definitely* too long.

By the time you start dialing in your long fast, you've already done one fasting day. Maintain a decent caloric intake the rest of the week, and then fast again on Sunday. Check your weight throughout the week, and see if your HGH boost has caused your weight loss to trigger.

If you're feeling really adventurous, throw another fast day in on Wednesday or Thursday. This will cause some pretty dramatic weight loss, but if you begin losing energy or muscle mass you've taken things too far. Resume the once-a-week fasting pattern.

If your standard caloric-restriction diet limits you to (say) 2,000 calories per day, it is perfectly acceptable and even recommended to continue maintaining a 2,000 calorie per day average over the course of the week. In other words, if your weight loss goal is 2,000 calories per day, you should translate that into (2,000x7=) 14,000 calories per week, and then divide it by the number of days in which you will be eating. In other words, consume 2,333 calories on your other days to make up for a one-day fast, or for the more extreme two-day fast, consume 2800 calories on the other five days.

Remember, the idea here is to replicate Thag's feast-or-famine lifestyle, not to starve you into a state of skinniness. You still want to hit all of your caloric goals; you're simply moving around the times you eat with the times you don't.

The Short ("Daily") Fast

Was the twenty-four hour fast just too much for you? Did you wake up Monday morning and savage a pig with your bare teeth, so ravenous were you?

Well, don't despair; you're not going to be a long-faster, and that's perfectly fine. Your cycle's a bit quicker than the twenty-four hour fast allows, and there's nothing wrong with that.

Again, the whole goal is calibration.

Happily, many of the benefits of fasting can still be yours. For you, though, the goal will be keeping your daily caloric intake goal, but limiting the time of the day in which you can eat.

We'll do this by leveraging your natural fasting period: overnight.

Consider for a moment the word "breakfast." The origin of that word should be clear if I spell it just slightly differently: "break-fast." Even in the old days, it was understood that going to bed at night began a fast period. In order to set a short, daily fasting schedule we're simply going to not break that fast.

Instead, find a period of time in the afternoon/evening that works for you. A common starting fasting schedule is the 16/8 fast, which begins at 8:00 pm and runs until noon the next day, with a feeding window between noon and 8:00 pm.

More extreme is the 20/4 fast, which gives you only a four hour window (say, from 1-5pm in the afternoon, or from 4-8pm in the evening) in which to consume your calories.

Don't try to break your fast in the morning, and then begin it at noon. To begin with, this pattern requires you to be awake for your endorphin-withdrawal hunger, while beginning the fast while you're asleep allows you to sleep right through that torturous period. Furthermore, the most effective hours of the fast are the last ones; that's when the body has kicked itself into lethal-machine mode. Spending *that* time asleep doesn't leverage the calorie-burning potential of your fast.

Whatever the window, remember that your caloric intake should remain the same. The goal here *is not starvation*. It is simply to reallocate one's timing of caloric intake to take advantage of Thag's established hormonal systems.

The nice thing about the daily fast is its consistency; you are able to establish a daily routing and follow it. Once it becomes a pattern, it becomes easy to follow. Fasting isn't an event like it is in the long-fast format; it's simply what you do every day. This kind of patterning makes it easier to stick with.

Of course, if you're a long-fast person there's no reason you can't perform some limited short-fasting on the days you do consume calories. This sort of mix-and-match diet can have powerful results. Just remember to keep your overall caloric intake in line with your recommended weight loss goal, and you'll be good.

Exercise and Fasting

For years, we have been inundated with commercials about "fueling up" for exercise. Of course, it's very hard to sell us nothing, and very easy to sell us energy drinks, energy bars, and any number of other gimmicky products.

The fact is, though, that fueling up for a workout is kind of a bonehead move. "Fueling up" here is simply a reference to caloric intake; the idea of fueling up before a workout is to consume calories, and then burn those calories during a workout. The problem, of course, is that we don't *want* to consume *those* calories during a workout; the goal of the workout should be to consume the calories our bodies have locked up in our fat.

Thus, the most effective workouts we can have are during our fast periods. While we're on (say) the popular 16/8 fast schedule, it's much more effective for us to work out in the morning, *during* our fast period. Our body has no food to burn during this phase, and is *forced* to reach down into our fat to fuel our workout. Therefore, while consuming BCAA or some other protein supplement prior to your workout is perfectly fine, don't "fuel up." The goal here is to run your primary tank on empty so that you burn your reserve fuel instead.

Trust, but Verify

Once you've got your fasting schedule, stick with it. Continue to monitor yourself. This is not a crash diet, and *it should not produce crash diet results.* If you find yourself losing, say, 8-10 pounds in a week, you have gotten something terribly wrong. You're likely consuming muscle mass, and that's not what you want.

That said, if you've judged your overall caloric intake correctly, you should experience steady, maintainable weight loss. Keep monitoring yourself, but if you find yourself losing 2-3 pounds a week and still feeling energetic, then welcome to the Intermittent Fasting lifestyle!

It's a Lifestyle, Not a Fad!

At the end of the day, dieting is some pretty straightforward math. You have your RMR, you have your caloric intake. Line the two of them up. If your RMR is greater than your caloric intake, you lose weight.

So many fad diets try to complicate that math.

Your basic fad diet goes something like this: "Eat X servings of Y calorie type at precisely 12:36 pm in order to cleanse the toxins from your liver, then consume A amount of B food type at precisely 1:47 in order to increase the functionality of your Whatsit. After that, take C number of these *special super vitamin supplements* that I have sold to you at $20.00 per bottle in order to catalyze your thingamajig."

Ok, I may be exaggerating, but only slightly.

If you've been on the diet rollercoaster long enough, you've seen countless diets like this, and none of them have actually worked. Now you're here, and you've picked up this book. You're staring at these words, looking at the eating patterns and the promises of weight loss, and there's decent odds you're feeling a little bit jaded.

After all, this is just another fad diet, right?

Well, it's not. To begin with, this isn't a diet in the strictest sense; it's a lifestyle. It isn't about *what* to eat; your calorie goals remain in place. It's about *when* to eat it.

More than that, though, this isn't a diet based on some obscure Mediterranean culture, or Ancient Taoist Wisdom, or some other such hokum. This is a return to our primal roots. Ancient Wisdom has nothing to do with it. I can think of a lot of descriptors for our good friend Thag, but wise is not one of them. This isn't about Ancient Wisdom, it's about ancient necessity, and the evolution that came about because of it.

And it has produced scientific results.

The idea that intermittent fasting is a new fad should be simply discarded here, because scientific testing on it began in 1913. Back then, the testing was largely on animals, but the overall consensus was that a pattern of intermittent fasting caused an extended lifespan.

Since then, we've been able to come up with several reasons why. Scientific testing continues today and the results seem to be pretty darn conclusive.

Remarkable Health Benefits

When Dr. John Berardi began his self-experimentation with the intermittent fasting lifestyle, he settled on a combined daily-fast pattern with a single long-fast in a week.

He reported successful, sustained weight loss of twenty pounds, lowering his weight from one hundred ninety pounds to one hundred and seventy pounds over the course of a month and a half, and then maintaining that one hundred seventy pound mark for over four months.

This is in line with what other studies show us; caloric restriction without under-nutrition produces consistent, stable weight loss. Intermittent fasting is a successful method of performing caloric restriction without under-nutrition.

Where this becomes interesting is that we are not talking simply about *weight loss,* but about *fat loss.* In his self-experimentation, Dr. Berardi noticed a drop in his body fat from ten percent to four percent. That means in the loss of only twenty pounds, he dropped more than half of his body fat. While Dr. Berardi was not exactly out of shape to begin with, that kind of targeted weight loss, burning away the fat and leaving the muscle mass intact, provides for a kind of overall fitness that simple caloric restriction simply does not match.

It is the kind of weight loss we all long for, the kind of weight loss promised by every fad diet out there; the loss of fat and the appearance of muscle.

What's not to love there?

Craving reduction

I've covered this before, but it's worth noting that this sort of intermittent fasting comes with a built-in control mechanism. By centering our natural, psychological hunger craving patterns to while we are asleep, it reduces the craving for food we feel 4-5 hours after a meal.

This allows us to stay on track with our diet more easily.

The fact of the matter is, it is this craving that eventually destroys most dieters. The constant, nagging pressure in the back of your head chanting at you to eat, eat, eat continues to force your psychological stress levels ever upward.

That kind of stress only goes away when you finally break down in an avalanche of pizza, ice cream, and self-loathing.

Obviously, we want to avoid that sort of a break, and intermittent fasting provides us that trick; when we go to bed, our voice has not begun its insistent chant. By the time we wake up, our voice has starved to death, leaving us free to restrict our calories how we will. The overwhelming conclusion of researchers is that intermittent fasting reduces the food cravings felt by dieters simply on a caloric restriction diet.

Insulin Stability

Welcome to 21st century America, the land of diabetes. The American Diabetes Association estimates that 8.3% of the population of America have diabetes. Of those, almost a third are undiagnosed.

America is a country whose blood sugar has run totally out of control. That's not surprising; think of the number of sugar-laden products that are presented to you on a daily basis. Soda? Candy? Just about anything cooked at a fast-food joint? We have a sweet tooth in this country, and it's been kicking the daylights out of our pancreases.

Diabetes is, of course, a disease in which the pancreas ceases to effectively regulate blood sugar through the production of insulin. Insulin is, if you will, the anti-sugar, the thing that keeps sugar in check.

Back in the day, Thag really didn't have access to that much sugar. Digging up a camas root would have given him a little starch; finding some berries at the right time would have given him a bit of a sugar buzz, but his diet simply didn't involve a high sugar count. What sugar he got, he got irregularly.

As a result, guess what Thag's system adapted to do? If you guessed "adapted to regulate spikes in blood sugar but not constant intake," then you've been paying attention.

You see, like many drugs, the human body can develop a tolerance toward insulin. (ADA) If you constantly spam your body with sugar, then your pancreas is constantly spamming your body with insulin. Eventually, your body becomes tolerant of the insulin, making it less and less effective.

That's type II diabetes in a nutshell; prolonged and ingrained resistance to insulin.

Which is why an intermittent fasting diet is so interesting. By having long periods of time in which your blood sugar is low, you also have extended periods of time when your pancreas gets to take a rest; you don't need all that insulin running about. Since you're on less insulin, you become less tolerant of the insulin. It becomes more effective.

In fact, a 2005 Copenhagen study tested this. It checked after only fifteen days of an intermittent fasting regimen, and found that insulin levels really hadn't statistically changed, but the rate at which that insulin was dealing with blood sugar had showed a marked increase.

What does this mean? It means that, even assuming you don't change *what* you eat, simply changing *when* you eat it may result in a significantly reduced chance of developing type II diabetes.

Heart Health

Weight loss is, of course, going to lead to a healthier heart. However, that's not the only part of intermittent fasting that has a cardiac benefit.

Once again, Thag's system comes into effect. His heart wasn't built to pump food-based nutrients about all the time; it's built to do that at sporadic intervals. Thag's entire body was designed to cope with intermittent fasting, and his heart was certainly no different.

Even accounting for all other factors (weight, blood sugar levels, diet), the stress patterns intermittent fasting places on the heart have been shown to lower coronary arterial disease by up to 12%.

I'll say that again, because it bears repeating: Simply by changing the time at which one eats, one has a 12% better chance of avoiding a coronary. Add to that the increased heart health from weight loss and avoiding diabetes, and you've got a really substantial cardiac benefit to the intermittent fasting lifestyle.

Increased Lifespan

I'm getting skinnier and healthier on this diet; doesn't that naturally lead to a longer lifespan?

It does, but there's more to it than that.

Remember somatotropin, the human growth hormone? It has a direct effect on aging. While the peer-reviewing jury is currently out on HGH supplements or shots, we know that HGH produced in one's own body is directly correlated to natural lifespan.

Directly correlated to natural lifespan.

Higher HGH levels cause rejuvenation of the body's tissues; joints become less sore, muscle mass increases, and *organs rebuild easier.* That means any method by which we can increase our *natural* HGH levels is going to increase both the length of our lives as well as the quality of those lives.

Now, we know that intermittent fasting increases HGH levels. HGH is the hormone that caused Thag to become a killing machine when it was time to hunt his next bison; it's stimulated by periods of fasting.

So, yes. Weight loss will lead to a longer life. The lack of diabetes will lead to a longer life. The lack of heart disease will lead to a longer life. But independent of all of those, the increase in your HGH levels will also lead to an extended natural life span.

To sum up, intermittent fasting causes better health through weight loss, diabetes prevention, heart health, and HGH production. This sounds like we're in the too-good-to-be-true category, but it only makes sense.

Remember, intermittent fasting isn't new; it's simply a return to the way our bodies were designed to cope with food. In that light, *of course* it's better all the way around.

The Journey of One Thousand Miles

Biology is, in the end, a pretty amazing thing. It has granted us a deep complexity. The number of systems our bodies have, the chemicals being secreted, the bacteria in symbiosis, the muscles and organs and bones, all of it is such a delicately balanced thing.

Each system relies upon the other, and has evolved into higher, more complicated, more delicate forms.

From that balance, we live.

Our caveman Thag, of course, never really thought about biology beyond finding just the right spot to hit a bison with a spear. The idea of insulin counts or human growth hormone never consciously crossed Thag's mind. But even though he never chose to consider it, he was setting the patterns for our bodies.

When Thag had food, he feasted. When Thag didn't have food, he was in famine.

The modern world is just not built around that kind of a cycle. Most of us go through our entire lives without having to kill our food. Even our present day hunters, though, use guns or (at the worst) finely calibrated bows to kill their food; there's no chasing down a bison with a spear for them. For plants, we farm; Thag would spend days looking for edible roots.

But mostly, we pull into the drive-thru windows of the local Fast Food joint. We send out for pizza. We microwave burritos and we open our refrigerators to find a variety of fruits, vegetables, and meats inside that would, frankly, have blown Thag's mind.

If we spend an hour cooking dinner, we think we've worked for it.

By caveman standards, an hour of daily cooking would be luxurious. Our farmers know what the best roots are (carrots, beets, potatoes, onions), and what's more we've found out that dipping them in boiling oil makes them even more delicious. We've also learned to extract sugar and fat from plants and animals, and we can just add those things to other foods.

It's not hard to imagine a simple guy like Thag being overwhelmed by the products available to us in the modern world.

What this book has tried to impress upon you, above all else, is that we *are* Thag in many, many ways. Our minds and our culture may be leaps and bounds above our caveman ancestors, but our bodies are no different.

The next time you look at your breakfast plate with its eggs, bacon, and toast, imagine that your body is Thag's body. It's overwhelmed by the abundance of food, and it isn't working right. It's making you hungry all the time, even when you don't need to be. It's shutting down its production of HGH. It is producing insulin on overdrive, and your heart is needlessly working overtime.

Your body is not built for the way you've been raised to treat it.

Three meals a day is simply a cultural evolution. Mealtimes are polite, social times. That structure grew out of our cultural desire to share food, and our desire to show off with food.

Our three-square-meals-a-day is something we are raised to believe is healthy, but there's little biology behind it. Such a myth should fall into the same category as treating a cold with chicken soup or candling wax out of your ears.

By not respecting the way Thag lived his life, we take the finely-tuned machine that is our bodies and destroy it. We pour gas into a diesel engine, and wind up with similar results.

Every system that relies on our digestive system to operate gets thrown just a little out of whack, like putting a weight on a single blade of a helicopter. Intermittent fasting has been referred to as a fad diet, but that's just risibly far from the truth.

It wasn't a fad diet for Thag; it was simply the way the world worked. It wasn't a fad diet for Thag's body; *it was simply the way the world worked.* Our modern diet, with its abundance, its decadence, and its rotting convenience, is the fad by comparison.

This book is here to encourage you to return to the simple way the world used to work.

Don't think of intermittent fasting as a fad diet, and don't treat it like a crash diet. It's not a race to see how long you can go without food, and it's not there to shape up for swimsuit season and then stop. Intermittent fasting is a lifestyle change, and one that, when applied correctly, can help to drastically improve both the length and quality of your life.

By taking a page out of our distant ancestor's book, we can restore that delicate formula and get our bodies back to the finely-tuned balance that Thag and his bison-chasing put them into in the first place.

Lao Tsu tells us that a journey of a thousand miles begins with but a single step. Well, our journey is not a thousand miles; it's fifty thousand years in the past. Regardless, now is the time to take that step.

We'll keep the electric lighting and the antibiotics, but our patterns of eating need to get back into the ancient ways.

Our basic, primal nature simply demands it.

Next Saturday, note the time you have dinner. On Sunday, skip the eating; just little snack before bed. See how you feel on Monday.

Your journey toward this ancient, healthier lifestyle will have begun.

Additional Resources

Calorie King Calculator:

http://www.calorieking.com/interactive-tools/weight-maintenance-calories-calculator/

This awesome free calculator lets you enter your gender, height and weight to get a relatively accurate estimate of how many calories you're currently burning in a single day. Use this number as a baseline guide when estimating how many calories you've cut from your diet.

Fast Food That Won't Kill You:

http://www.fitnessmagazine.com/recipes/healthy-eating/on-the-go/healthy-fast-foods/

This article in Fitness magazine outlines 24 not terrible fast food options from KFC, McDonald's, Taco Bell, Wendy's and Pizza Hut. Having a few semi-healthy options in mind can be a huge help if you find yourself in a social situation where fast food is the only option. For example, did you know that

Taco Bell's Chicken Gordita with Nacho Cheese only has 270 calories? Order two of those and you've got a 540 calorie meal that won't destroy your day or make you feel like you're "on a diet" when you're out with friends. Compare that to the Taco Bell Fiesta Taco Salad, which clocks in at a surprising 860 calories and you'll see why it's smart to know a few decent options for each fast food chain. Just in case.